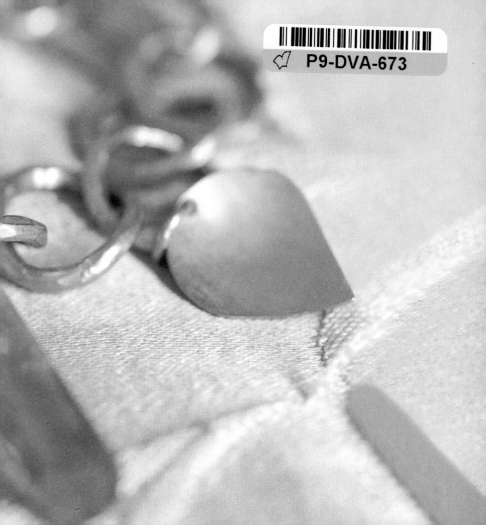

# *A PASSION FOR*

# CHARMS

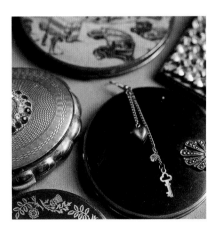

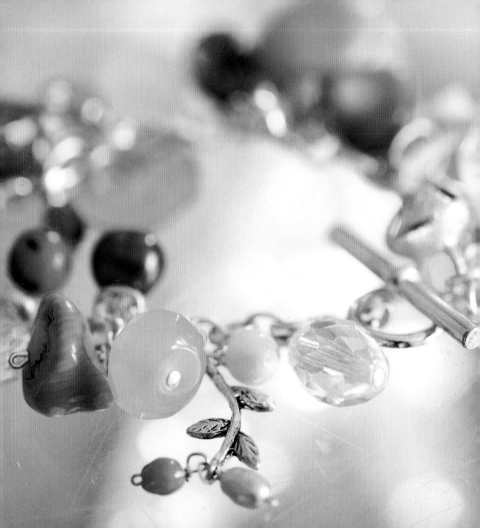

# *A PASSION FOR*
# CHARMS

**Amy Elliott**
photography by **Sandra Lane**

RYLAND
PETERS
& SMALL
LONDON NEW YORK

Designer  **Pamela Daniels**
Commissioning editor  **Annabel Morgan**
Location researcher  **Tracy Ogino**
Production  **Gemma Moules**
Art director  **Anne-Marie Bulat**
Publishing director  **Alison Starling**

Stylist  **Lorraine Dawkins**

First published in the United States
in 2006 by Ryland Peters & Small
519 Broadway, 5th Floor
New York, NY 10012

10 9 8 7 6 5 4 3 2 1
Printed in China

ISBN-10: 1-84597-264-3
ISBN-13: 978-1-84597-264-6

Library of Congress cataloging-in-
publication data has been applied for.

# contents

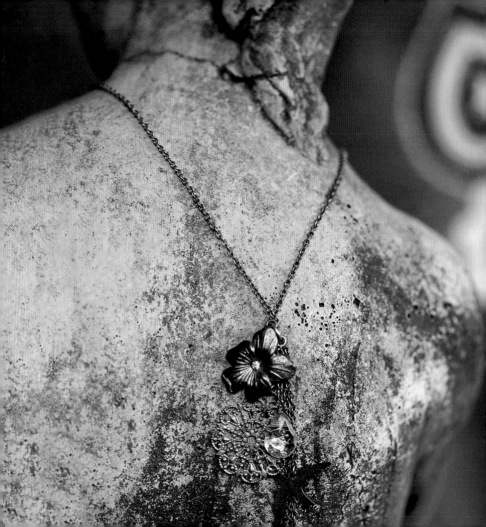

# introduction

Charms are fashionable again, and you don't just see them on bracelets. They dangle from chains and ribbons like little clusters of grapes; they swing from hoop earrings and designer handbags, and even loop round the slender stems of wine glasses at dinner parties. Your charm bracelet or necklace may be a gem-studded piece worthy of wearing to a black-tie event, or karmic and mystical, all Om symbols and crystals. Meanwhile, your friend's bracelet may be strictly sentimental, bearing a tiny trinket for each baby's birth and a gold heart for every wedding anniversary.

What's behind the current revival of interest in charms? Perhaps it can be linked to an influx of ladylike clothes on the runway, from Hitchcock-heroine tweeds and cashmere sweaters, to ruffled chiffon tea dresses and demure blouses embellished with lace. As stylish as they now are, charms are still the storytelling, heirloom treasures they've always been. My hope, as you peruse the pages of this book, is that you'll be encouraged to rediscover any charm bracelets you might own, unearthing them from the bottom of a dressing-table drawer,

*"Adornment is never anything except a reflection of the heart."*

COCO CHANEL

*Vivienne Westwood, Chanel, Marni, Louis Vuitton, Burberry, Dolce & Gabbana, Banana Republic, Lulu Guinness, and Juicy Couture have all produced charm bracelets (or belts, necklaces, and earrings).*

or the velvet-lined depths of an old jewelry box. (And you can always consider swiping your mother's or grandmother's if you haven't got one of your own!). Alternatively, you may be inspired to start collecting charms for the very first time, or to create a charm bracelet that reflects your own individual passions, hobbies, and interests.

When it comes to seeking out new charms, the most droll and fascinating ones are usually vintage, and the best place to hunt for these is at flea markets, antique stores, and estate sales. Contemporary charm jewelry is sold at local jewelry stores, over the internet, and at some of the world's most glamorous jewelry houses. And you can turn to the sources listed on page 63 for a few ideas to start with.

Whether you wear charms to be chic, to express yourself, or as a superstitious safeguard against danger, you're certain to find more than a few ideas in this little book. So go on—look, learn, and luxuriate in the charming world of charms.

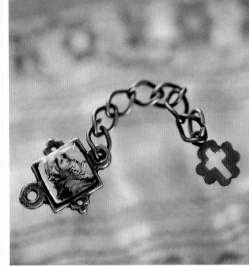

*"Chunky gold bracelets with handsome baubles or charms of semiprecious stones are amusing and chic..."*

FROM *A GUIDE TO ELEGANCE* (1964),
BY GENEVIEVE ANTOINE DARIAUX

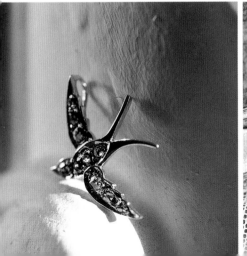

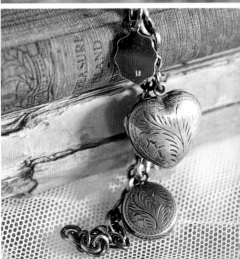

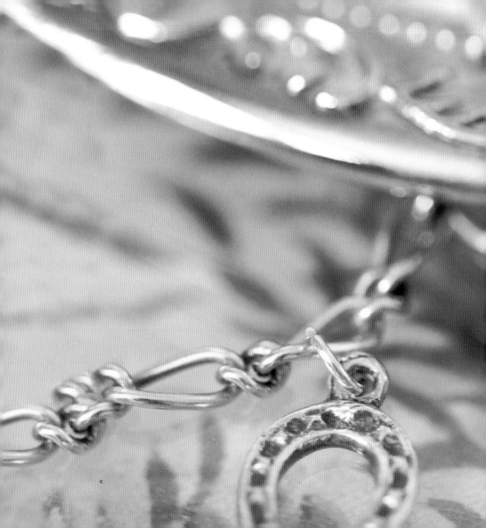

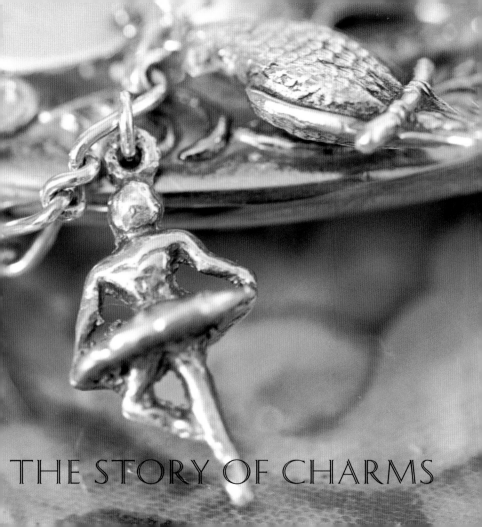

THE STORY OF CHARMS

# the first charms

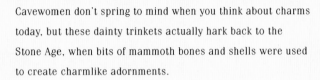

*Historically, men were the first charm-wearers— they wore their jewelry as a status symbol and as good-luck amulets to aid them in battle.*

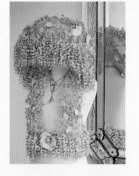

Cavewomen don't spring to mind when you think about charms today, but these dainty trinkets actually hark back to the Stone Age, when bits of mammoth bones and shells were used to create charmlike adornments.

The Babylonians are thought to be the first civilization to have worn charms on a bracelet, while the ancient Egyptians wore charms to attract good luck and protect them from evil spirits. The Egyptians were also highly skilled goldsmiths and paved the way for future generations of jewelry designers. In the Middle Ages, charmlike medallions were worn to indicate social status. And Renaissance-era monarchs and aristocrats were rarely seen in public without piling on luxurious pendants embellished with rubies, emeralds, and pearls.

Today, most of us wear charms the way our 19th-century ancestors did—to be fashionable, to express our tastes, and to record our experiences. And this "charming" tradition will hopefully continue to be passed down through the ages and enjoyed by future generations.

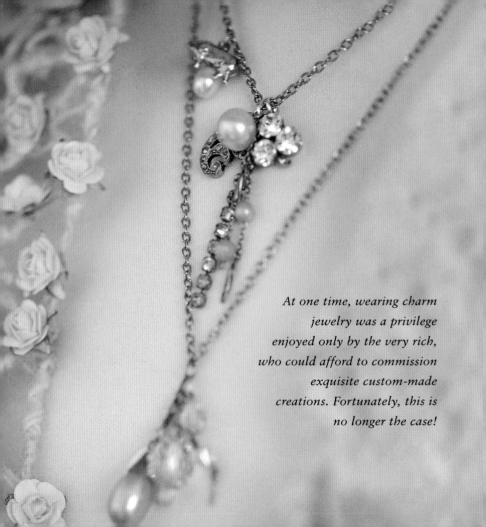

*At one time, wearing charm jewelry was a privilege enjoyed only by the very rich, who could afford to commission exquisite custom-made creations. Fortunately, this is no longer the case!*

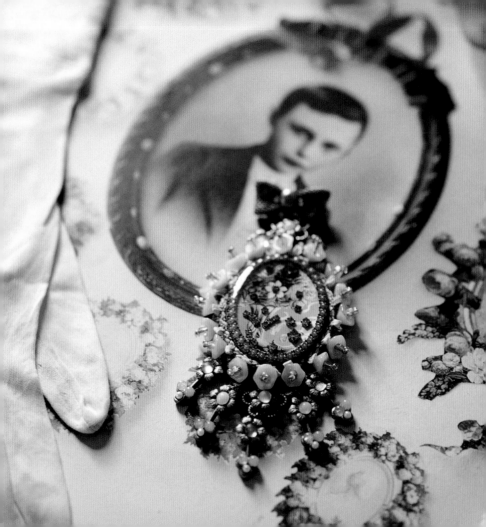

# the victorian era

*The Victorians were coy when it came to expressing their emotions. They used charms to convey a coded message: for example, a bracelet with diamond, emerald, amethyst, and ruby charms, spells out D-E-A-R, using the first letter of each gem.*

Modern charm-wearers owe a great deal to Queen Victoria (1837–1901), one of the most romantic monarchs in history, whose collection of charms and trinkets ignited a trend that has never gone out of fashion. Her fabulous jewels and tiaras are legendary, as is her penchant for sentimental jewelry—she wore miniature portraits of her nine children on a gold bracelet, while a miniature portrait of her beloved Prince Albert dangled from a bracelet made of pearls.

Thanks to Victoria's example, lavish ornamentation, particularly with sentimental jewelry, became de rigueur during the Victorian era. It was considered fashionable, for example, to wear "hair jewelry"—bracelets, necklaces, and earrings that incorporated a loved one's locks. Elegant Victorian ladies also favored cameo brooches worn as pendants on velvet ribbon. Whimsical birds, insects, and flowers, often set with coral, amethysts, and seed pearls, or wrought in intricate combinations of gold and enamel, were all popular charm motifs during this period.

# *contemporary charms*

Charms exploded onto the scene with new vitality during World War II. Throughout this period, charms were produced in mass quantities and at all price levels, from patriotic charms in the Tiffany & Co. catalog to cheap plastic good-luck charms you could enclose in a love letter to your sweetheart overseas. But the trend really took off when the soldiers came home, bringing charms they had picked up during their adventures in Europe and the South Pacific.

The 1950s marked the charm bracelet's heyday, when it became an all-out obsession, a symbol of femininity itself. Popular movie stars like Elizabeth Taylor, Lucille Ball, and Natalie Wood cast charm bracelets in a glamorous light every time they were photographed wearing them. Meanwhile, many a suburban woman kept house and mixed cocktail-hour martinis with a bracelet flashing dainty charms for culinary skills, a green thumb, or the birth of a child on her wrist. Later, this same woman would create charm bracelets for her daughters, who wore them in the 1960s until it was no longer considered "cool" to do so.

Fast-forward to today, and we're in the midst of yet another charm-bracelet craze. Hip girls have turned them into high-fashion accessories, or sport their mother's or grandmother's in an ironic nod to the conventions of yesteryear.

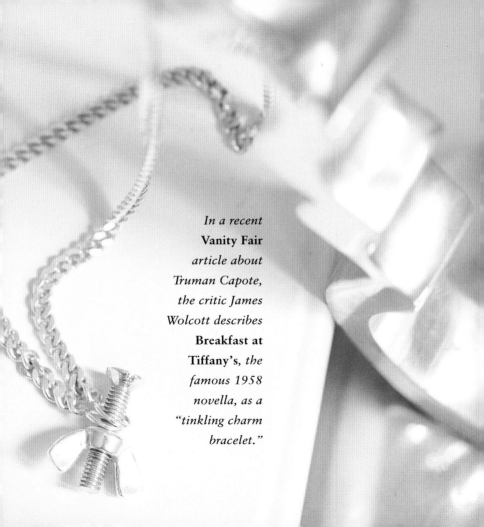

*In a recent* **Vanity Fair** *article about Truman Capote, the critic James Wolcott describes* **Breakfast at Tiffany's,** *the famous 1958 novella, as a "tinkling charm bracelet."*

they wr

distracted

wn elevatio

vlity and purity be

se

# TOKENS OF AFFECTION

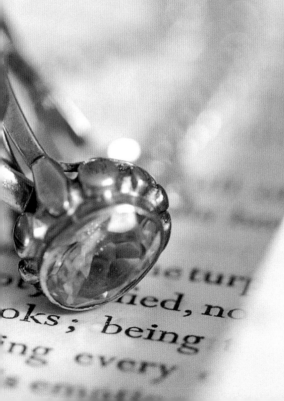

# *"I love you" charms*

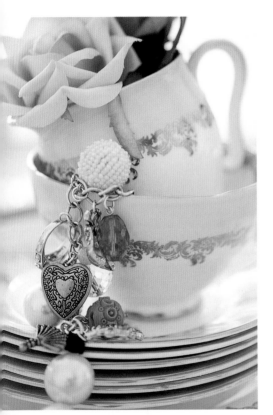

When jewelry is used as a symbol of passion and devotion, love is a many-splendored thing indeed. Charms have always been a popular and eloquent way to express the heart's emotions.

Some charms playfully hint at pet names and private jokes, while others are purely sentimental. A gilded picnic basket can pay tribute to a first date or a little laptop computer can commemorate a relationship that blossomed online, while a do-not-disturb sign conjures up happy memories of lazy honeymoon mornings spent in bed.

Whether they are dangling from a bracelet or suspended around the neck, charms are so romantic that receiving one will make any girl melt with delight.

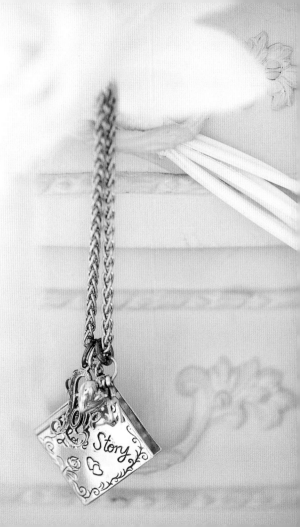

*"Heart charms always signify a great emotional connection. The oldest ones I ever acquired were from 1870, five gold and diamond hearts, each engraved with a different child's birth date, and given by a husband to his wife."*

CAMILLA DIETZ
BERGERON, ESTATE
JEWELRY DEALER

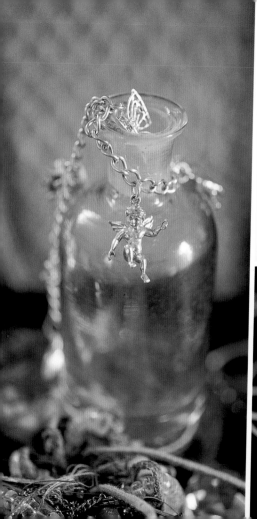

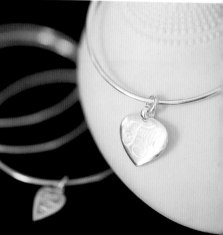

*"God save the King for Wallis
16.VII.36"*

INSCRIPTION ON THE BACK OF A
CROSS PENDANT BELONGING TO WALLIS
SIMPSON. IT WAS GIVEN TO HER BY PRINCE
EDWARD, BEFORE THEY WERE MARRIED,
TO ADD TO VARIOUS OTHER CROSS
CHARMS SHE WORE ON A BRACELET.

Personal inscriptions and engravings make an intimate gift even more meaningful. The nature of these markings range from simple and heartfelt: "To Joan, all my love" (to actress Joan Crawford from actor Franchot Tome when they were a couple); to cryptic: "We'll see" (to the founding editor of *Cosmopolitan* Helen Gurley Brown from one of her suitors) to downright hilarious: "I'm sorry" (to an Average Jane, on the back of a doghouse charm displaying a photo of the offending Average Joe).

Other ideas include a meaningful quote, such as "A queen in crown of rubies drest" (taken from "To The Same Flower" by William Wordsworth), or more intriguing inscriptions, such as "115" (referring to one couple's shared love of a particular Shakespeare sonnet), or even "34.04N, 118.15W" (being the latitude and longitude of where one couple met and fell in love).

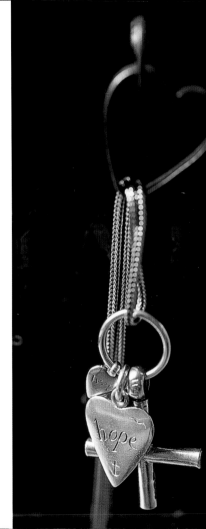

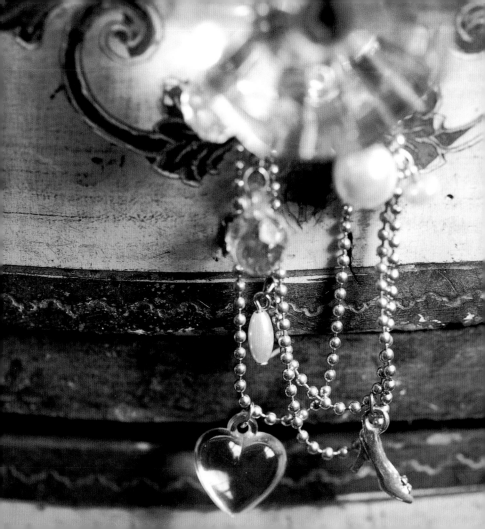

# hearts

Cupids, the Chinese "Double Happiness" character, "X"s and "O"s, a serpent biting its tail. All these objects symbolize affection, but none capture the essence of romantic love quite as perfectly as a heart-shaped charm. Heart-shaped baubles can be gem-studded and showy, simple and inscribed, or as humble as a plastic heart from a box of Cracker Jacks.

How did the heart shape come to be so closely associated with all things romantic? It's actually an aesthetically pleasing version of the anatomical organ, said to be the dwelling place of our deepest emotions. It's no secret that feelings of love can trigger a physiological reaction in the heart.

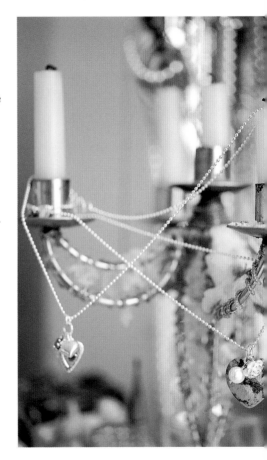

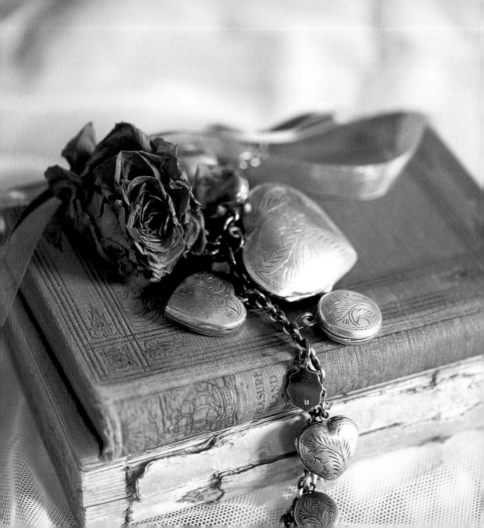

# lockets

*"The next thing to catch her eye was...a gold locket, and opening this she was startled indeed; for it contained a portrait in miniature of the gallant youth she had seen in her dream."*

FROM *BEAUTY AND THE BEAST*, BY SIR ARTHUR QUILLER-COUCH

Few of us would burst into tears upon receiving a heart-shaped locket from Tiffany & Co. but that's exactly what happens in the Broadway musical *Annie*: Daddy Warbucks gives one to the heroine, Little Orphan Annie, telling her that he wants to adopt her, and Annie weeps because she already has half a locket. Her birth parents left it with her when they dropped her at the orphanage, and kept the other half, promising to come back for her one day. Naturally, it would be impossible for a shiny new locket to trump her sentimental attachment to the one she already owns!

Many other little girls, and women, have a similar affection for their lockets, traditionally a hinged pendant, often heart-shaped, that's used to encase a photo or a lock of hair. Lockets enjoyed widespread popularity during the Victorian era (the jewelry-loving queen herself owned several), and today they remain among the most loving gifts you can give or receive—perfect for children, bridesmaids, new mothers, and sweethearts alike.

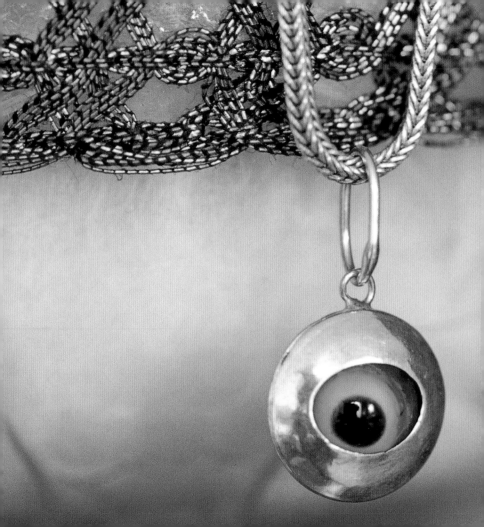

# GOOD-LUCK CHARMS

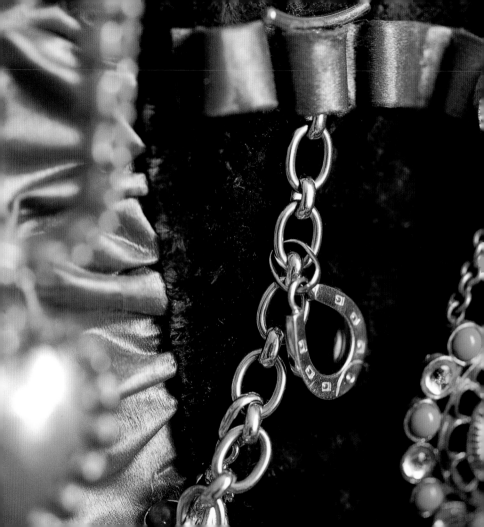

# *lucky charms*

*The legendary Coco Chanel was mad for symbols, including "5," her lucky number, thanks to the success of her best-selling fragrance, Chanel No. 5.*

Originally, charms were thought to possess magical powers, promising long life, luck, and prosperity to those who wore them. How does an object or image become lucky? A combination of old wives' tales, religion, and ancient mythology. Countless amuletic charms are available today, their mystical properties still believed by many to be effective. As you shop for charms, keep an eye out for these:

THE FOUR-LEAF CLOVER is one of the most ubiquitous symbols of good luck. Its leaves represent hope, faith, love, and luck.

LAUGHING BUDDHAS are an Asian symbol of good luck, but you don't have to be a Buddhist to reap the benefits. According to legend, if you rub a buddha's belly, your chances for good fortune will increase significantly.

JADE, apple-green, smooth, and glossy, is another traditionally Asian amulet that is believed to cure disease and is carried to attract joy and prosperity. Jade is particularly sacred to the Chinese, who believe that the stone embodies all of the "Five Virtues": charity, modesty, courage, justice, and wisdom.

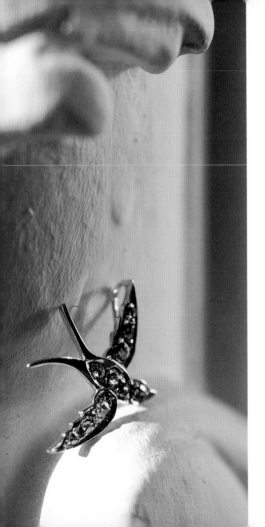

ELEPHANTS are considered lucky because of Ganesh, the elephant-headed Hindu god of wisdom, dignity, and prosperity. When selecting an elephant charm, make sure its trunk is tilted up, not down— otherwise, your luck will run out!

GOLDFISH symbolize wealth and prosperity (imagine a goldfish charm set with yellow diamonds or sapphires—stunning!).

LADYBUGS are always auspicious, especially if they land on you. In charm form, make sure your ladybug has lots of spots, because the more there are, the luckier you'll be.

GAMBLING CHARMS. Jeweled dice, gold poker chips, or tiny packs of playing cards are sure to keep you in Lady Luck's good graces.

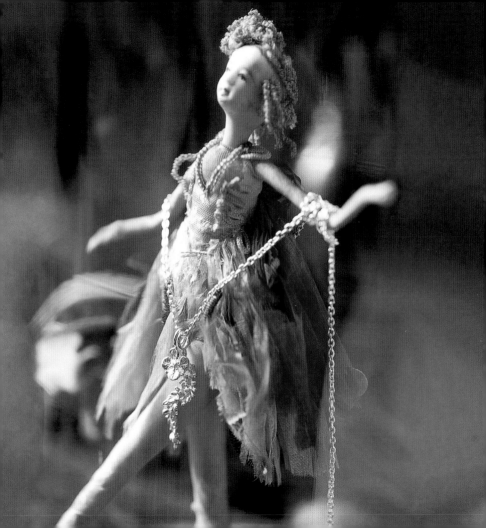

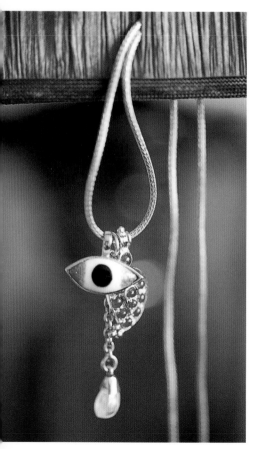

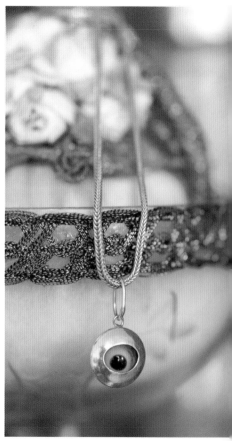

# *protection against evil*

*Just to be on the safe side, many women wear heaps of evil eye bracelets at one time. The eyes typically feature blue irises with black pupils, and are made of glass.*

While some charms are worn in the hopes of attracting good luck, others are believed to protect the wearer from life's most malevolent pariahs—financial loss, sickness, marital troubles, and other unwelcome situations. Consider wearing any of the charms below, if only for good measure:

A HORSESHOE is a powerful protective talisman, thanks to the old-fashioned tradition of nailing a horseshoe above the entrance of a house, to shield both the structure and its inhabitants from witches, Satan, and other malicious evil-doers. Accordingly, wearing a horseshoe charm on a bracelet or necklace (always with the prongs up, so the good luck doesn't drain away) offers a girl the same form of protection when she's out and about.

THE EVIL EYE emerged as a menace in many ancient and medieval cultures—if someone gave you the "evil eye" (a mean-spirited, envious, or foreboding glare), it was believed that you'd meet with the worst kind of misfortune. The evil eye amulet, which resembles an eye (see pictures on left), operates on the "fight-fire-with-fire" principle: if the evil

*Consider a charm made of red coral for little girls— it's said to protect children from injury and disease. Of course, you can get one for yourself, too— coral is a protective amulet, promoting mental clarity and emotional stability.*

eye's gaze should be directed at you, your evil eye amulet will (hopefully!) ward off the onset of bad luck.

THE HAND OF FATIMA is a charm that averts the "evil eye" in Middle Eastern and Jewish cultures. A hand with three downward-pointing fingers and two thumbs, modern versions sometimes feature semiprecious stones, and often display elaborate engraving or filigree details.

SCARABS are representations of dung beetles, which were revered by the ancient Egyptians as a symbol of resurrection and immortality. Often carved from soapstone, amber, turquoise, and other semiprecious materials, scarabs offer you protection in this life, and in the afterlife.

Other protective charms you might like to add to your charm collection include the horn, which looks something like a long red chili pepper, and jingling bells, which have a long history of warding off evil spirits.

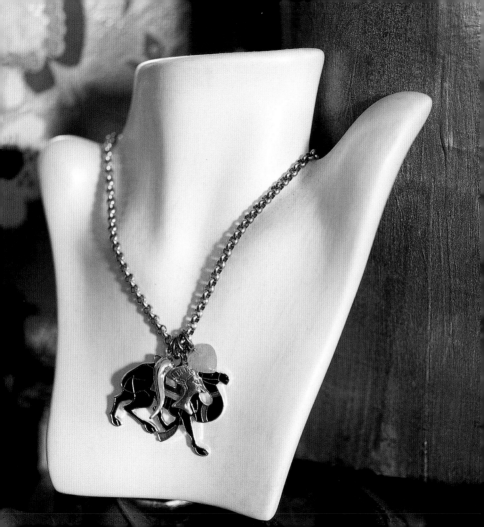

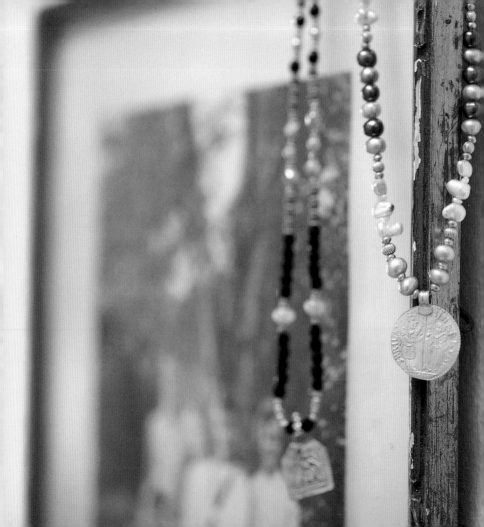

## *tiny treasures*

With their shiny luster and intricate details, even the humblest penny looks charming on a necklace or bracelet. Gold coins in particular are associated with wealth and happiness and are considered inherently lucky. Bracelets made entirely of coins were popular in the 19th and early 20th centuries; later Coco Chanel gave coins pride of place in many of her costume jewelry collections.

Contemporary jewelry designers continue to be inspired by coins, including Tamsin de Roemer, whose pieces are featured in the photograph on the left. Here, antique coins displaying Indian deities (traditionally worn for protection) are suspended from necklaces fashioned from pearls and semiprecious stones.

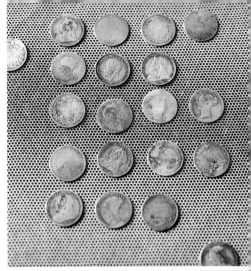

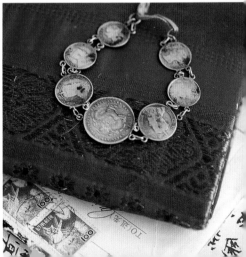

# *birthstones*

*Is it bad luck to wear opal if it's not your birthstone? No! This superstitious myth surfaced in the 19th century because of a popular novel by Sir Walter Scott. Queen Victoria helped to reverse the negative connotation by wearing opals in abundance and by giving opal jewelry as gifts.*

Precious and semiprecious gems have long been associated with curative and mood-altering powers; each one possesses its own unique attributes. Everyone has a birthstone, so don't be shy about letting anyone who might give you a gift know what yours is! Birthstone charms, like a pansy with amethyst petals, or a fairy with emerald-studded wings, are very symbolic, for all gems have special properties.

JANUARY Garnet (loyalty, friendship)

FEBRUARY Amethyst (wisdom, peace)

MARCH Aquamarine (tranquility)

APRIL Diamond (strength, everlasting love)

MAY Emerald (fertility)

JUNE Pearl (purity, innocence)

JULY Ruby (passion, joy)

AUGUST Peridot (friendship, charity)

SEPTEMBER Sapphire (fidelity, truth)

OCTOBER Opal, (hope)

NOVEMBER Topaz (true love)

DECEMBER Turquoise (success, good fortune)

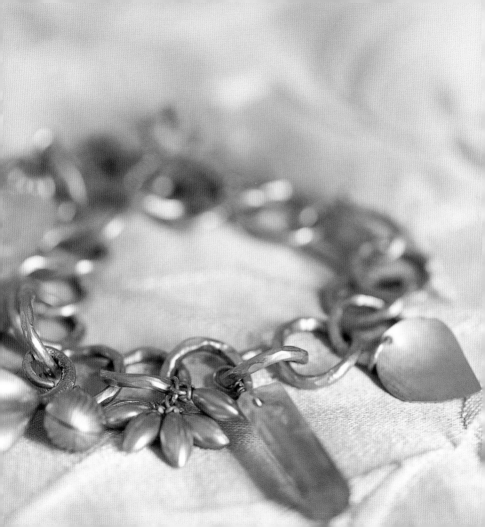

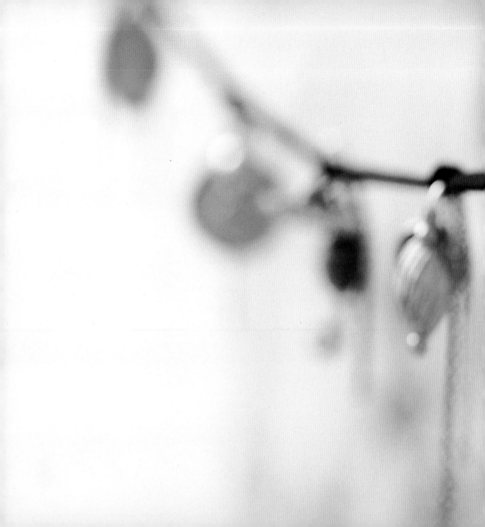

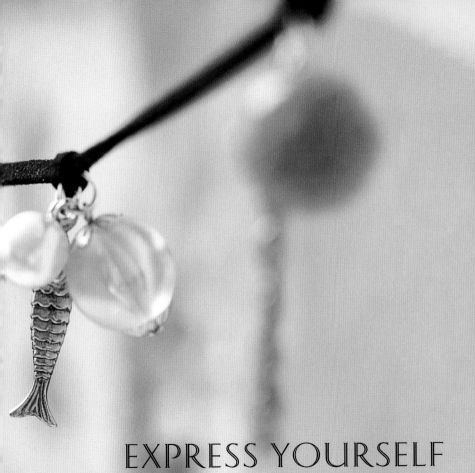

EXPRESS YOURSELF

# *hobbies and interests*

Binoculars for a bird-watcher. Trainers for a marathon runner. A tube of lipstick or a martini glass for a party girl. Each item pinpoints someone's favorite passions and pastimes, and makes a perfect gift—especially if they appear in the form of a miniature gold or silver trinket.

"Many of the best charm bracelets are those built around people's unique lives and interests," says Lisa Slutsky, co-owner of C.H.A.R.M., a New York City jewelry design firm that specializes in sourcing unusual vintage charms. "One of our clients had just bought a country house, so we made her a bracelet that exemplified her idea of the perfect home. We used 35 charms, including a lightbulb, a coffee grinder, a vacuum cleaner, garden shears, and even a little chihuahua."

Rebecca Wynnewood, a librarian living in New York City, is fond of her mother's charm bracelet, which includes tiny ballet slippers, a pair of ice skates ("for when she learned how to skate at Wollman Rink in Central Park," says Rebecca), and a gold tennis racquet accented with a tiny

*"We sell a great deal of toilet bowl charms at Christmas time. I hope this just means there are a lot of plumbers out there!"*

JENNIFER HILLMAN,
COMMUNICATIONS
DIRECTOR,
REMBRANDT CHARMS

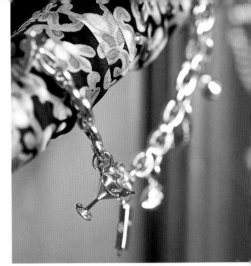

*"My ultimate charm bracelet would include vintage pieces: diamonds, pearls, colored pieces, and small icons including hearts, shoes, bags, umbrellas, and sunglasses. I love 1950s motifs which are humorous but also elegant."*

LULU GUINNESS,
ACCESSORIES DESIGNER

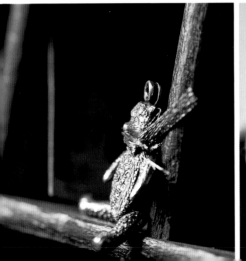

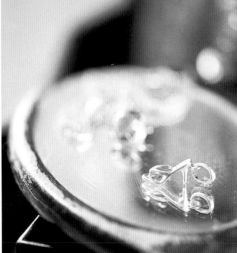

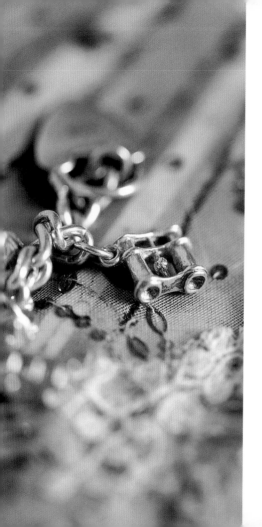

pearl tennis ball. "I'm adding my own charms that reflect my love of books and New York history," she says.

While "favorite thing" charms can be playful, even a bit bizarre (how about a corncob pipe?) they can also be quite elegant. Anne Barge, a wedding gown designer based in Atlanta, Georgia, says that, in addition to fashion, she's always been interested in music and the arts. "As a teenager, I had a beautiful gold artist's palette charm with ruby, sapphire, and emerald dollops of paint," she says. "I also had a grand piano charm with sapphire and ruby keys."

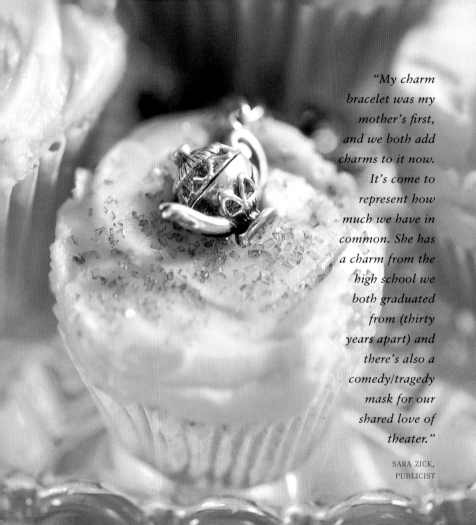

"My charm bracelet was my mother's first, and we both add charms to it now. It's come to represent how much we have in common. She has a charm from the high school we both graduated from (thirty years apart) and there's also a comedy/tragedy mask for our shared love of theater."

SARA ZICK,
PUBLICIST

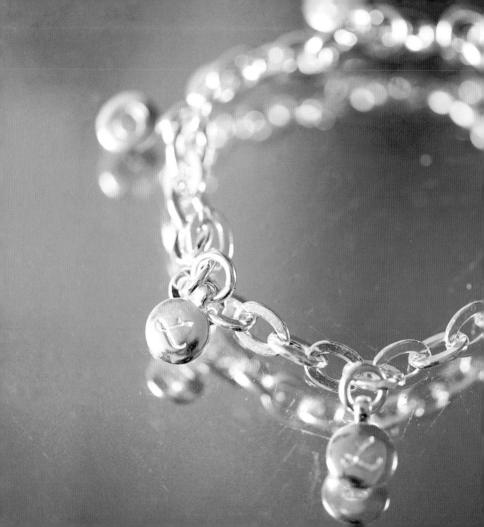

# *monograms and initials*

What's the easiest way to make your charm bracelet even more personal? Have a charm engraved with your monogram. If a trio of interlocking letters isn't your style, most jewelers will have several typefaces and designs to choose from.

Monogrammed jewelry is a throwback to medieval heraldry, when elaborate coats-of-arms, emblazoned on a shield, or worn in pendant or insignia form, indicated your ancestry and rank. Hundreds of years later, the inclination to wear a bauble that identifies you still remains. Personalized pendants recently enjoyed a huge resurgence in popularity, perhaps due to Carrie Bradshaw (Sarah Jessica Parker's *Sex and the City* character) wearing a nameplate necklace. Others think the emotional fallout following September 11th rekindled a fondness for trinkets linked to family traditions.

Today, it's chic to wear single-letter charms: a diamond "A," or a "V" engraved on a silver disc. Consider wearing two on the same bracelet or chain—your first and last initials, or a coy combination of you and your sweetheart's first initials.

*"Unless a crest is being used, a monogram—or initials—is the best marking, and the best number of letters is three. (Two or four are perfectly correct but difficult to work into a pretty design.)"*

FROM *VOGUE'S BOOK OF ETIQUETTE* (1948), BY MILLICENT FENWICK

# *moments and milestones*

If charms don't reflect a woman's hobbies and interests, then they usually mark an important event in her life. Sweet-sixteen birthdays, graduations, weddings, and anniversaries are certainly all charmworthy occasions, but baubles that celebrate the birth of a child seem to be the most popular by far. "The most important jewelry I own is related to significant moments in my life," says the Italian jewelry designer Silvia Damiani. "When my son Leonardo was born, I received a beautiful pendant from one of our collections. It looks like a big strawberry made of sapphire and diamonds. I love it because it's chic, but it's also cute, like a toy."

Hollywood moms, such as Jennifer Garner, Reese Witherspoon, and Kate Beckinsale love designer Helen Ficalora's dainty "Alphabet" charms, which lend themselves particularly well to birth jewelry. "The charms display a single letter on a gold disc, and new moms like to wear their children's first initials on a chain, sometimes along with their own," says the designer, whose own "family necklace" includes her first initial, as well as her sons' and husband's.

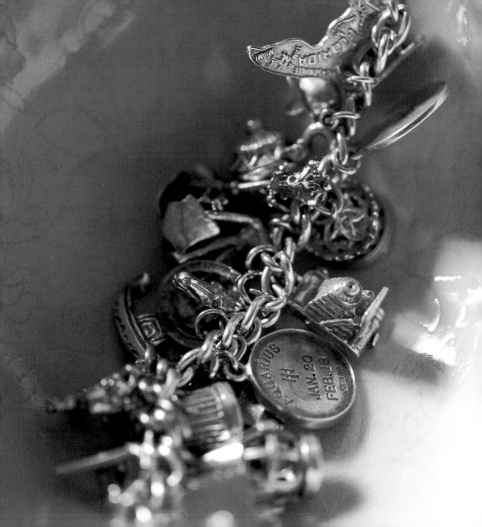

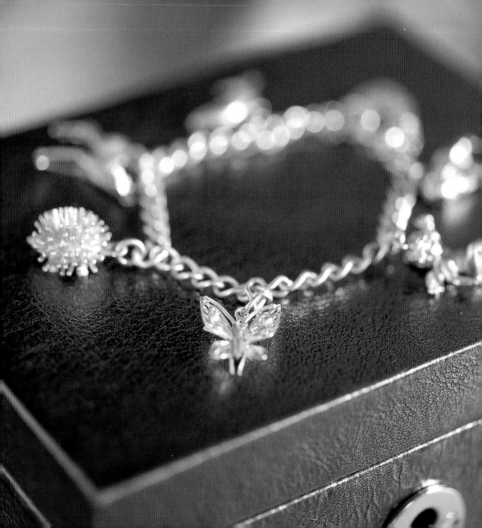

## *dream up a theme!*

There's something quite captivating about a jumble of mismatched charms on a bracelet, but it's also clever to assemble a group of tokens with an underlying theme. Two ideas to try:

### THE "BIRTHDAY" BRACELET

(let's say yours is May 30th): A Gemini charm, a charm (or several!) accented with emerald (May's birthstone), the number 18 (21, 30, 40 and so on, according to which milestone birthdays you've reached), a birthday cake, and a bottle of champagne.

### THE "I LOVE SUMMER" BRACELET

A lemonade stand, a jeweled flip-flop, a starfish, a straw sunhat, a seashell, a lighthouse, a seagull (or a pink sapphire flamingo!), and an ice-cream cone.

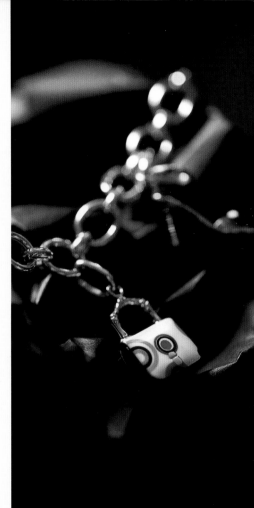

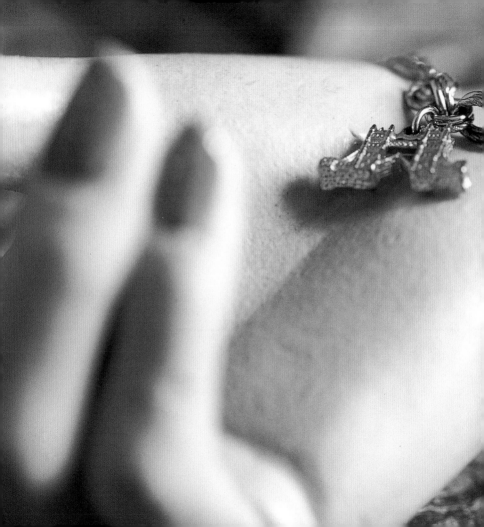

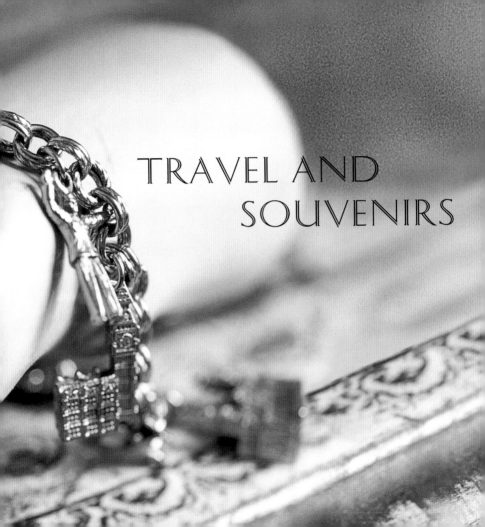

TRAVEL AND
SOUVENIRS

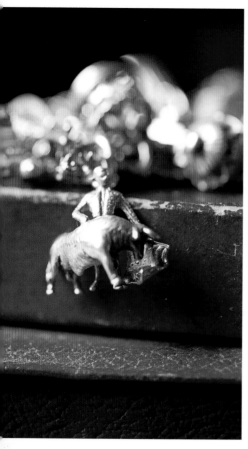
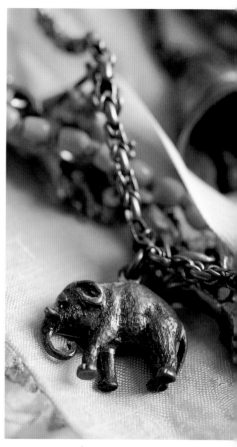

# *charming adventures*

While some charms indicate who you are and what you love, travel charms whisper of where you've been and what you've experienced. For most of us, the instinct to gather and preserve tangible memories of our travels is innate, whether we're harvesting pebbles and seashells from a beach, or pocketing matchbooks, metro passes, and ticket stubs to paste in a scrapbook. Grand tours and spontaneous getaways are always well-represented on charm bracelets—a silhouette of the state of Florida, a miniature Arc du Triomphe, or a black pearl pendant from Tahiti are souvenirs that have an almost magical ability to transport the owner back to a special time and place.

*"Throw off the bowlines, sail away from the safe harbor. Catch the trade winds in your sails. Explore. Dream. Discover."*

ATTRIBUTED TO
MARK TWAIN

Charms like passports, airplanes, and "Bon Voyage" pennants are sometimes given in anticipation of a big trip. And globetrotting parents frequently gift their charm-collecting daughters with little trinkets from the destinations they've visited. But the most common souvenir charms are the ones you pick up yourself. Laurel Cardone, a copy-editor in Brooklyn, New York, wears a striking gold charm bracelet

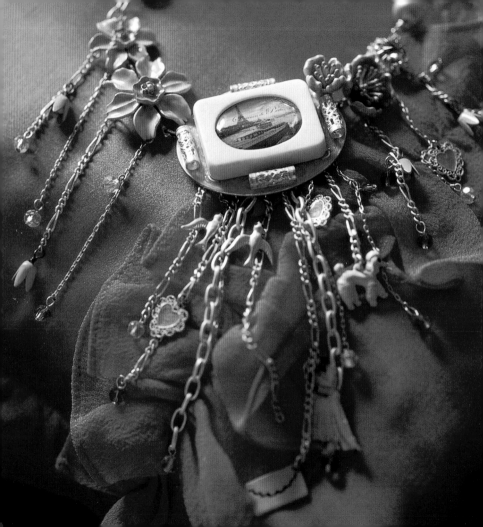

with a lone gold coin dangling from one of the links. "It's a coin from Aruba, and my parents bought it while on their honeymoon in 1964," she says. "My mother used to wear it on a chain around her neck, and now I wear the charm on a bracelet that once belonged to my father. I love the sentimentality of it."

Serious charm collectors are always on the prowl, whether they're at a yard sale down the street, in a jewelry store on Madison Avenue, or trolling the stalls of a Moroccan bazaar. But plenty of travel charms are purchased from local jewelers after the event. While on holiday, why not jot down the landmarks, images, and foods that leave an impression on you, so that you can shop for charms when you get home?

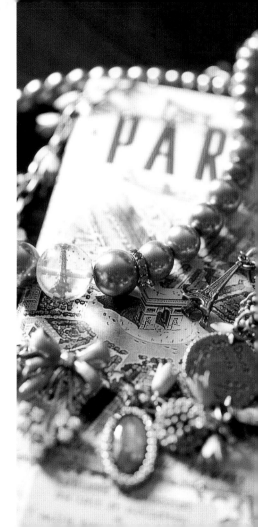

## safe passages

Carolyn Rafaelian, of the Rhode Island-based jewelry design firm Alex and Ani, recently created a bangle bracelet with a St. Christopher charm on it—proceeds were donated to families affected by Hurricane Katrina.

Some travel charms serve as protective amulets to finger, or even bring to your lips, when the plane ride gets bumpy, or if you should find yourself lost and bewildered in a big city. The St. Christopher's Medal—usually a gold disc depicting a benevolent-looking man with a child held aloft on his shoulders—is the most famous of these.

St. Christopher, originally called Offero, was a giant-sized man of superhuman strength whose job was to carry travelers safely across a treacherous stream. One day, he carried a child who seemed to get heavier and heavier. The child explained that this was because he had the weight of the world on his shoulders; revealing himself as Jesus Christ, he baptized Offero on the spot and gave him the name Christopher, which literally means "Christ-bearer."

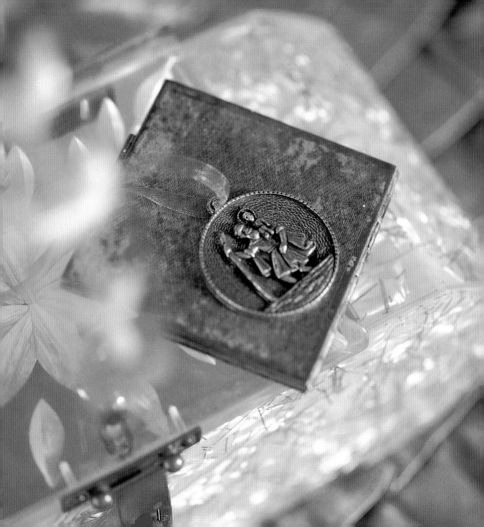

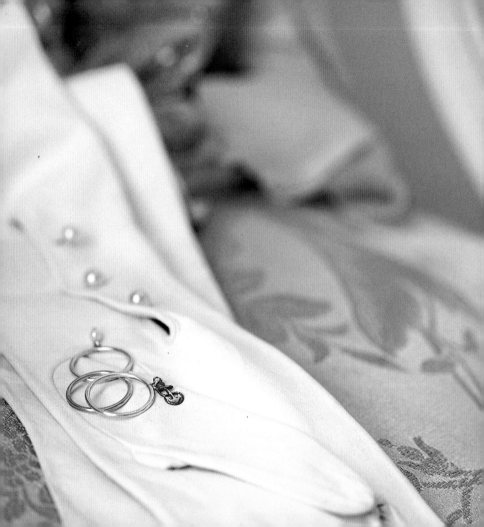

# sources and business credits

ALEX AND ANI
www.alexandani.com
*Funky charm jewelry for the
21st-century girl.*

AZUNI
www.azuni.co.uk
*Bracelets, silver charms, and
semi-precious stones.*

C.H.A.R.M.
www.charmco.com
*Striking antique and vintage-
inspired charms. Many
popular themes—the cute
beauty and fashion charms
include a gold stiletto heel,
a credit card, and even a
tiny hairdryer!*

DAMIANI
796 Madison Avenue
New York, NY 10021
212-375-6474
www.damiani.com
*Exquisite Italian fine jewelry
with some bejeweled charms.*

DE ROEMER
www.deroemer.com
*Coin charms and bold evil
eyes set in gold.*

CAMILLA DIETZ BERGERON
818 Madison Avenue, 4th floor
New York, NY 10021
212-794-9100
*by appointment only
Estate jewelry dealer.*

HELEN FICALORA
www.helenficalora.com
*Simple, elegant gold discs
stamped with the letters of the
alphabet and words such as
"mom," "love," and "smile."*

MARTE FRISNES JEWELLERY
www.martefrisnes.com
*Handmade bracelets inspired
by Marte's native Scandinavia.*

LULU GUINNESS
www.luluguinness.com
*Adorable bags and accessories.*

LINKS OF LONDON
www.linksoflondon.com
*Gold and silver charms.*

MAISONETTE
www.maisonette.uk.com

MARIANNE
+44 20 7435 2151
*Vintage home accessories.*

MAX OLIVER
+44 20 7354 0777
www.max-oliver.co.uk
*Luxury lifestyle boutique.*

PIPPA SMALL
www.pippasmall.com
*Bold and unique jewelry.*

PAUL SMITH
+44 20 7379 7133
www.paulsmith.co.uk

REMBRANDT CHARMS
www.rembrandtcharms.com
*Huge selection of gold and
silver charms. Visit their
website for details of your
nearest stockist.*

SALOON
+44 20 7278 4497
www.saloonshop.co.uk
*Accessories and vintage finds.*

V V ROULEAUX
www.vvrouleaux.com
*Exquisite ribbons.*

WRIGHT AND TEAGUE
www.wrightandteague.com
*Silver charm bangles and
bracelets, many inscribed.*

# *picture credits*

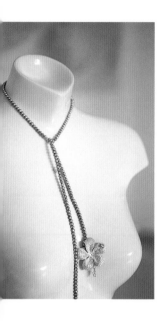

Key: a=above, b=below, r=right,
l=left, c=center

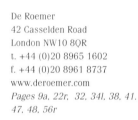

De Roemer
42 Casselden Road
London NW10 8QR
t. +44 (0)20 8965 1602
f. +44 (0)20 8961 8737
www.deroemer.com
*Pages 9a, 22r, 32, 34l, 38, 41,
47, 48, 56r*

Julia Clancey
www.juliaclancey.com
*Pages 12–13, 18–21, 25, 62*

# *acknowledgments*

I am indebted to author Ki Hackney, my amazing friend and mentor,
who first introduced me to the charm of charms.

I would also like to thank all the friends and designers who so generously
shared their charming stories with me, especially Jennifer Hillman at
Rembrandt Charms, Silvia Damiani, Helen Ficalora, Lisa Slutsky, Anne
Barge, and Ms. Lulu Guinness. Finally, thank you, Mom: your passion
for jewelry is always a source of amusement and inspiration.

The publishers would like to thank all those who allowed us to
photograph in their homes for this book, including Marianne Cotterill,
fashion and jewelry designer Julia Clancey, Ros Fairman, and Justin
Packshaw and jewelry designer Tamsin De Roemer.

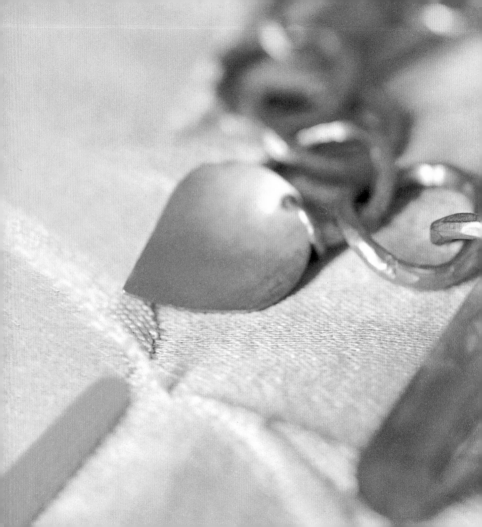